Other Works by This Author

Weapons Grade Moxie: Unleashing Your Inner Strength to Conquer Fear and Toxic People

Wholeness Through Illness- Finding Meaning, Healing, and Grace

You Are Infinite!: Co-Creating the Fractal Holograph

Unstuck: Experiencing the Anahata Nad

The Pineal Portal: Unlocking The Secrets of The Third Eye

Life In The Bliss Lane: A Guide To Wellness, Self-Love, And Joy

Killing Time: Breaking Free From Temporal Chains

Level Up With Gratitude: The Ultimate Bio-Hack For Happiness

Ardhanarishwara Charitra: The Metaphysical Wisdom of Gender Fluidity

Vasudhaiva Kutumbakam: The Limitless Power of Our Desi Roots

The Atma's Journey: Tarot Wisdom Through the Ramayana & Mahabharata

You Make Me Sick: Virtue Signaling & Narcissistic Abuse

Toxic Sibling Estrangement: Reclaiming Your Inner Peace

Hidden Branches In The Family Tree: Navigating the NPE Experience

Beyond Binary: An Exploration in Gender and Sexuality

Pharmajuana: Guide to Cannabis for Cancer

Why Straight Lines Don't Exist: Exploring Geometric Truths

How to Gym: Becoming Fitness Itself

P.E.A.K.: Phenomenological Experiences At Kailash

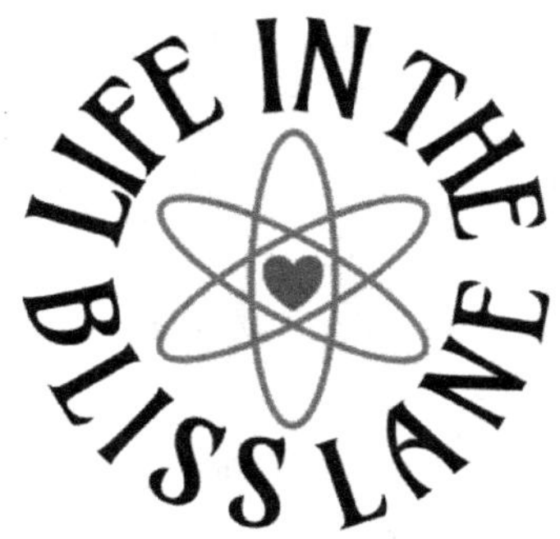

Life in the Bliss Lane

Copyright ©2024

For Agni

You got this.

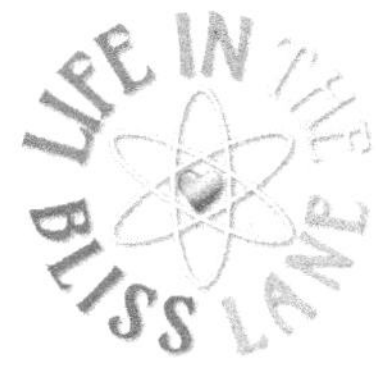

INTRODUCTION

UNDERSTANDING THC: A Guide for Cancer Patients

In the evolving landscape of medical cannabis, tetrahydrocannabinol, or THC, stands out as a beacon for its potential therapeutic benefits, especially in the realm of cancer care. As you navigate through your treatment journey, understanding the different types of THC can empower you to make informed decisions about incorporating cannabis into your health regimen. Let's demystify the various forms of THC and explore how they can be tailored to meet your unique needs.

PHARMAJUANA

NAVIGATING LEGAL LANDSCAPES: A RESPONSIBILITY FOR PATIENTS

As the landscape of cannabis legalization continues to evolve globally, the legal status of cannabis, both for medicinal and recreational use, varies significantly from one region to another. This book focuses on the medical applications of cannabis in the treatment of cancer, providing insights into how different types of cannabis can be used to manage symptoms and potentially affect the course of the disease. However, it is beyond the scope of this book to delve into the specifics of cannabis legality in various jurisdictions.

UNDERSTANDING YOUR RESPONSIBILITY

Stay Informed: It is crucial for patients considering cannabis as part of their cancer treatment to stay informed about the laws in their specific area. Legalities surrounding cannabis can change frequently, and what may be permissible in one state or country can be illegal in another.

Consulting Professionals: While this book provides a medical perspective on the use of cannabis, patients should also seek advice from legal professionals or local authorities to understand the specific regulations applicable to them. This is particularly important when acquiring, possessing, or using cannabis to ensure full compliance with local laws.

Accessing Safe and Legal Cannabis: Patients need to ensure that any cannabis they obtain for medical use is sourced through legal and safe channels. This not only ensures compliance with the law but also guarantees that the cannabis is of high quality, free from contaminants, and safe for medical use

WHY LEGALITIES ARE NOT ADDRESSED IN THIS BOOK

Regional Variations: The global landscape of cannabis legalization is highly fragmented. Detailed legal advice relevant to one locality might not apply to another, making it impractical to provide specific legal guidance that would be universally applicable or useful.

Focus on Medical Information: The primary aim of this book is to educate cancer patients and healthcare providers about the potential medical benefits of cannabis, including its therapeutic effects and how it can be integrated into cancer care. Addressing legal issues would require a different focus, potentially detracting from the medical advice and patient support that is the core purpose of this text.

Legal Expertise: Legal advice should be given by qualified professionals who specialize in local cannabis regulations. This ensures that patients receive the most accurate and up-to-date information pertinent to their specific circumstances.

PHARMAJUANA

CONCLUSION

As you consider incorporating cannabis into your cancer treatment regimen, it is imperative to be proactive about understanding the legal framework in your locality. This responsibility lies with each patient and their support network to ensure that their use of cannabis is not only effective and safe but also fully compliant with local laws. By focusing on the medical aspects of cannabis use within the framework of existing regulations, this book aims to provide valuable insights while encouraging lawful and informed decision-making.

PHARMAJUANA

A SACRED LEAF: THE TIMELESS MEDICINAL USE OF CANNABIS AROUND THE WORLD

Cannabis has been revered as a medicinal herb across various cultures for millennia, earning the euphemism "God's Own Medicine." This term underscores the plant's simplicity and natural efficacy—no preparation is required to tap into its healing powers, suggesting a divine intent for its use. This chapter explores the rich history of cannabis as a sacred medicine, tracing its journey through ancient civilizations to its continued veneration today.

ANCIENT BEGINNINGS

China: The medicinal use of cannabis dates back to ancient China, around 5000 years ago. The Chinese emperor Shen Nung, considered the father of Chinese medicine, documented the plant's properties in pharmacopeias, noting its effectiveness in treating ailments such as gout, rheumatism, and malaria. Cannabis was regarded as a symbol of yin, or feminine energy, and was used to balance various bodily systems.

India: In India, cannabis has been a sacred herb for thousands of years, integral to the religious and cultural fabric of the country. It is associated with the Hindu deity Shiva, who is said to have rested under a cannabis plant and consumed its leaves. Traditional texts like the Atharva Veda praise the plant as one of the five sacred plants that relieve anxiety. Cannabis continues to be used in religious ceremonies and Ayurvedic medicine, where it is prescribed for pain relief, stress reduction, and digestive disorders.

MIDDLE EASTERN AND AFRICAN TRADITIONS

Middle East: Historical records from ancient Assyria and Egypt show that cannabis was used for its psychoactive and therapeutic properties. The Ebers Papyrus, one of the oldest complete medical textbooks from Egypt, circa 1550 BCE, mentions cannabis as a medicine for inflammation and pain.

Africa: Cannabis spread to Africa, where it was used for a variety of medicinal purposes, including easing childbirth, treating malaria, and as an antiseptic. African tribes also valued cannabis for its psychoactive properties during religious ceremonies, believing it could facilitate communication with the divine.

EUROPEAN USE AND THE SPREAD TO THE AMERICAS

Europe: Cannabis was introduced to Europe during the medieval period. It was used in folk medicine for treating tumors, coughs, and jaundice. During the Renaissance, cannabis was studied by herbalists and botanists, further integrating it into Western medicine.

PHARMAJUANA

Americas: With the colonization of the Americas, cannabis was brought over by the Spanish and Portuguese. It was cultivated primarily for its fibers, but medicinal uses were documented in texts from the 18th century, noting its applications for treating skin burns, easing pain, and reducing fever.

MODERN REDISCOVERY AND REVERENCE

In the 19th century, Western medicine rediscovered cannabis, leading to a resurgence in its use for various ailments, from muscle spasms to chronic pain. It was during this time that the term "God's Own Medicine" likely gained popularity, reflecting its wide range of applications and minimal need for processing.

Today, the reverence for cannabis as a medicinal plant continues, supported by modern research into its therapeutic compounds. Legalization movements across the globe reflect a rekindling of the ancient trust in cannabis's healing properties, affirming its role as a natural, divinely inspired remedy.

CONCLUSION

The historical and ongoing medicinal use of cannabis across diverse cultures attests to its potent healing properties and sacred status. As "God's Own Medicine," cannabis is celebrated not only for its effectiveness but also for its natural origin, ready to be used as it is found. This deep, historical reverence informs contemporary attitudes and the legal landscape surrounding cannabis, as more people rediscover its benefits and integrate this ancient herb into modern medical practices.

PHARMAJUANA

THE DEMONIZATION OF CANNABIS: POLITICS, PROFIT, AND PREJUDICE

In this chapter, we explore the tumultuous history of cannabis in the Western world, particularly in America, where a confluence of political, business, and social factors led to its demonization in the mid-20th century. This section aims to uncover the insidious reasons behind the stigmatization of cannabis and highlight how this has deprived many, especially disabled individuals, of a potent therapeutic tool in their health arsenal.

ORIGINS OF STIGMA

The Early 20th Century: Cannabis began to face public and governmental scrutiny in the early 1900s in America, influenced by racially charged narratives and economic interests. The influx of Mexican immigrants during the Mexican Revolution of 1910 brought with it the recreational use of cannabis. The term "marihuana" was popularized in the U.S. to associate the plant with these immigrant communities, framing it as a source of social vice and criminal behavior.

THE MARIHUANA TAX ACT OF 1937

Political and Business Interests: The Marihuana Tax Act of 1937 marked a significant turning point. Lobbied by powerful figures such

PHARMAJUANA

as Harry Anslinger, head of the Federal Bureau of Narcotics, and supported by industries threatened by hemp (like cotton and paper), the legislation effectively criminalized marijuana. Anslinger used a campaign of misinformation and sensationalist stories in the media to paint cannabis as a dangerous drug that led to insanity, criminality, and death. This law was not scientifically driven but was influenced heavily by racial prejudices and economic interests aiming to remove hemp as a competitor in the textile and paper industries.

POST-WAR PARANOIA AND THE WAR ON DRUGS

Further Criminalization: In the decades following the Act, cannabis continued to be portrayed negatively as part of broader cultural and political conservatism. The 1950s and 1960s saw it associated with anti-establishment movements, which only intensified its demonization. The Controlled Substances Act of 1970 then classified cannabis alongside heroin and LSD as a Schedule I drug— defined as having a high potential for abuse and no accepted medical use, stifling further research and use in treatment.

IMPACT ON MEDICAL USE

Suppression of Information: The classification of cannabis as a Schedule I drug had dire consequences for medical research. With cannabis relegated to the same category as much harder drugs, the potential for its clinical application was largely ignored, and the development of cannabis-based treatments was halted. This suppression of information meant that when individuals, especially those disabled, were diagnosed with cancer, they were unaware of cannabis as a viable option for symptom management and treatment.

THE MODERN RECKONING

A Shift in Perception: It wasn't until the late 20th and early 21st centuries that the perception of cannabis began to shift due to advocacy, scientific research, and an increased public understanding of its medical benefits. States began to legalize medical cannabis, acknowledging its utility in treating a wide range of conditions, including cancer, chronic pain, and neurological disorders. This shift has been part of a broader movement to correct the historical injustices associated with cannabis prohibition.

WHY THIS BOOK MATTERS

In writing this book, my goal is to illuminate the obscured history of cannabis and reintroduce it as a significant and legitimate form of medicine, particularly for cancer patients. The demonization of cannabis has left a legacy of ignorance and fear, which this book aims to dispel. By providing evidence-based information, we can empower patients, especially those disenfranchised or disabled, to make informed decisions about their health and advocate for their right to access all beneficial treatments. The journey towards acceptance and understanding of cannabis is crucial for ensuring that all patients can access the care they need, informed not by historical prejudice but by contemporary science and compassion.

PHARMAJUANA

PHARMAJUANA

CANNABIS IN CANCER CARE: A MULTIFACETED APPROACH

Cannabis has re-emerged in the medical community as a powerful ally in cancer care, offering a spectrum of benefits from potential anti-carcinogenic properties to symptom management. This chapter explores the mechanisms by which cannabis aids cancer patients, shedding light on its diverse therapeutic roles that enhance both quality of life and potentially impact cancer progression itself.

ANTI-CARCINOGENIC PROPERTIES

Apoptosis Induction: One of the most promising aspects of cannabis in cancer treatment is its reported ability to induce apoptosis—programmed cell death—in cancer cells without harming normal cells. Compounds in cannabis, particularly cannabinoids like THC and CBD, have been shown to trigger this process in various cancer cell lines, including breast, lung, and brain cancers. This selective apoptosis helps reduce the size and growth of tumors.

Inhibition of Angiogenesis: Angiogenesis, the process by which new blood vessels form, is crucial for tumor growth. Research has indicated that cannabinoids can inhibit angiogenesis, thus starving tumors of the blood supply needed to grow and metastasize.

Anti-proliferative Effects: Cannabinoids have also been observed to inhibit the proliferation, or rapid growth, of cancer cells. By slowing the rate at which cancer cells replicate, cannabis can potentially help control the spread of cancer within the body.

SYMPTOM MANAGEMENT

Anti-emetic Effects: Nausea and vomiting are common and debilitating side effects of chemotherapy. Cannabinoids, particularly THC, have been recognized for their anti-emetic properties and have been used in synthetic forms like dronabinol and nabilone to treat chemotherapy-induced nausea.

Pain Management: Cannabis is well-known for its analgesic properties. Both THC and CBD contribute to pain relief by interacting with pain receptors in the brain and throughout the body, offering an alternative to traditional painkillers, which can be ineffective or cause significant side effects for some patients.

Neuropathic Pain: Many cancer patients experience neuropathic pain due to nerve damage from chemotherapy or the tumor itself. Cannabis has shown potential in relieving this type of pain, where other medications may fail.

IMPROVEMENT IN QUALITY OF LIFE

Anxiety and Depression Relief: Dealing with cancer can take a significant emotional toll on patients, leading to anxiety and depression. CBD is particularly noted for its anxiolytic effects without the psychoactive highs associated with THC, helping patients manage stress and improve their mood.

Improved Sleep: Symptoms like pain and anxiety can disrupt sleep, further impacting health and quality of life. The sedative effects of certain cannabinoids can help improve sleep duration and quality, aiding overall recovery and well-being.

Appetite Stimulation: Cannabis, especially THC, has been shown to effectively combat the loss of appetite seen in cancer patients, helping them maintain their nutritional status and overall strength during treatment.

INTEGRATING CANNABIS INTO CANCER TREATMENT PLANS

The benefits of cannabis in cancer care are supported by a growing body of research, yet it remains a complex field with much left to explore. For many patients, cannabis offers a source of relief and a hope for recovery not just through its potential direct anti-cancer effects but also through its ability to alleviate some of the most challenging symptoms of the disease and its treatments.

As research continues and the stigma surrounding cannabis diminishes, its role in cancer care is likely to become more significant and refined. It is important for patients to consult healthcare providers knowledgeable in cannabis use to tailor treatments to individual needs, ensuring safe and effective use of this ancient yet re-emerging natural therapy. This chapter aims to empower cancer patients with knowledge, advocating for informed choices in their treatment options and fostering a better understanding of how cannabis can be integrated into their cancer care regimen.

PHARMAJUANA

THE MANY FACES OF THC

DELTA-9-THC: THE MAIN EVENT

Delta-9-THC is the star of the cannabis world, renowned for its potent effects and the quintessential "high" it provides. Found abundantly in marijuana, it's the component that has been most studied for its therapeutic properties. For cancer patients, Delta-9-THC offers significant relief from nausea and vomiting caused by chemotherapy. It's also excellent at stimulating appetite, helping combat the weight loss that many face during treatment. Available both in natural forms and as a synthetic compound (dronabinol), it offers flexibility in how it can be used.

DELTA-8-THC: THE GENTLE COUSIN

A bit less famous but no less important, Delta-8-THC offers many of the benefits of Delta-9-THC but with a softer touch. Its milder psychoactive effects make it a preferred choice for those who want relief without intense high sensations. The calming and pain-relieving properties of Delta-8 can be a solace for those going through stressful treatments, helping manage both physical and psychological discomfort.

PHARMAJUANA

DELTA-10-THC: THE LIGHT TOUCH

If Delta-9-THC is a sprint, then Delta-10-THC is a gentle jog. With even less psychoactivity than Delta-8, Delta-10 is celebrated for its ability to uplift and enhance alertness without overwhelming effects. For patients who need a mild stimulant and mood booster while navigating the challenges of cancer therapy, Delta-10 can be an excellent addition to their therapeutic arsenal.

THCA: THE RAW PRECURSOR

THCA is what THC looks like before it heats up. Found in raw and live cannabis, this non-psychoactive precursor turns into Delta-9-THC when decarboxylated (heated). For those exploring cannabis's benefits without the high, consuming raw cannabis might offer anti-inflammatory and neuroprotective benefits, helpful in managing the broader symptoms associated with cancer and its treatments.

THCV: THE SLIMMING STIMULANT

Distinct from its THC siblings, THCV is known for suppressing appetite rather than enhancing it. It might sound counterintuitive for cancer care, but for patients dealing with specific types of appetite-related issues or metabolic health concerns, THCV offers a unique approach. Moreover, its potential to help with diabetes management and reduce panic attacks can be particularly beneficial for maintaining an overall balance.

PHARMAJUANA

INTEGRATING THC INTO YOUR TREATMENT PLAN

Choosing the right type of THC involves more than understanding its effects—it requires considering your overall treatment goals, existing health conditions, and personal comfort with cannabis' psychoactive properties. It's essential to consult with healthcare professionals experienced in medical cannabis to tailor the right concoction for your needs. Always remember, each body reacts differently to cannabis, and what works for one patient may not work for another.

NAVIGATING LEGAL LANDSCAPES

Before you embark on your THC journey, it's crucial to navigate the legal landscape. Cannabis laws vary widely by location, and understanding these can help you access safe, legal options for incorporating THC into your cancer care plan.

CONCLUSION

THC holds a complex but promising place in cancer care. By understanding the different types of THC, you can better navigate your options and find the formulation that best supports your journey to recovery and well-being. Remember, you're not just a patient; you're a pioneer in your health journey, exploring new avenues to improve your quality of life during and beyond cancer treatment.

EXPLORING CBD

Cannabidiol, or CBD, is a remarkable compound from the cannabis plant that has captured the attention of the medical community and cancer patients alike. Unlike its more famous cousin THC, CBD does not produce a psychoactive effect, making it an appealing option for those seeking relief without the high. This chapter will guide you through the different forms of CBD, their potential benefits, and how they can be integrated into cancer care.

THE SPECTRUM OF CBD

CBD Isolate: The Purest Form

CBD isolate is the purest form of cannabidiol, free from other cannabinoids, terpenes, and plant materials. It's 99% pure CBD, offering a straightforward option for patients who are cautious about THC or other compounds in cannabis. For cancer patients, CBD isolate can be a source of relief from inflammation, pain, and anxiety without any concerns about psychoactive effects.

Full-Spectrum CBD: Whole-Plant Synergy

Full-spectrum CBD contains all the phytochemicals naturally found in the cannabis plant, including a trace amount of THC (usually less than 0.3%). This type harnesses the power of the whole plant, creating what is known as the "entourage effect," where the therapeutic benefits are enhanced by the synergistic interaction of the compounds. For those battling cancer, full-spectrum CBD can help manage pain, reduce inflammation, and alleviate stress, while potentially enhancing the immune response.

Broad-Spectrum CBD: The Middle Ground

Broad-spectrum CBD strikes a balance between isolate and full-spectrum products. It includes most cannabinoids and terpenes but without THC. This type is suited for patients who want the benefits

of the full entourage effect but without any THC in their system. It's especially beneficial for those who may have sensitivities to THC or concerns about drug testing but still wish to receive the broader benefits of cannabis extracts.

THERAPEUTIC BENEFITS OF CBD IN CANCER CARE

Pain Management

CBD is widely recognized for its analgesic properties, making it a valuable ally in combating the chronic pain that often accompanies cancer and its treatments. It interacts with the endocannabinoid system to reduce pain signals, providing a natural pain relief option that is less reliant on opioids.

Anti-inflammatory Effects

Inflammation is a common complication in cancer, contributing to pain, fatigue, and other symptoms. CBD's anti-inflammatory properties can help reduce these symptoms and potentially improve the overall quality of life for patients.

Anxiety and Depression Relief

Dealing with cancer can be incredibly stressful, leading to anxiety and depression. CBD has been shown to exert calming effects, which can help stabilize mood and improve mental well-being, making it easier for patients to cope with the emotional challenges of cancer.

Nausea and Appetite

While not as directly effective as THC in managing nausea and stimulating appetite, CBD can complement THC-based therapies to help regulate nausea and maintain a healthier appetite during chemotherapy.

Neuroprotective Properties

Emerging research suggests that CBD may have neuroprotective properties, which could be beneficial in managing chemotherapy-induced neuropathy, a painful condition caused by nerve damage from certain cancer drugs.

INTEGRATING CBD INTO YOUR CANCER TREATMENT

Consulting with Healthcare Providers

Before adding CBD to your treatment regimen, it's essential to consult with oncologists and specialists who understand cannabis medicine. They can help tailor a CBD regimen that complements your existing treatments and addresses your specific symptoms.

Legal and Accessibility Considerations

CBD is generally more accessible and has fewer legal barriers than THC, but its legal status can still vary. Ensuring that you source your CBD from reputable, legal suppliers is crucial to receiving high-quality, effective products.

CONCLUSION

CBD offers a versatile and gentle approach to managing the multifaceted challenges of cancer. With various forms available, from isolates to full-spectrum products, CBD can be tailored to meet the specific needs and preferences of cancer patients, providing comfort and support through a natural, plant-based therapy. Embracing CBD can be a transformative part of your journey, potentially easing the path through treatment and recovery with grace and resilience.

TERPENES IN CANNABIS: ENHANCING CANCER CARE

Terpenes, the aromatic compounds found in various plants including cannabis, play a crucial role not just in determining the plant's scent and flavor but also in enhancing its therapeutic effects. In the context of cancer care, understanding the specific benefits of different terpenes can guide patients in choosing the most appropriate medical cannabis to meet their treatment needs. This chapter explores the properties of key terpenes and their potential applicability to cancer symptoms and treatment side effects.

UNDERSTANDING TERPENES

Terpenes are volatile organic compounds produced by many plants, and they are the primary constituents of essential oils. In cannabis, terpenes interact with cannabinoids (like THC and CBD) to potentially enhance the medicinal effects of the plant, a phenomenon known as the "entourage effect." This synergistic interaction can affect how cannabinoids bind to their receptors, impacting the overall efficacy and experience of cannabis.

PHARMAJUANA

KEY TERPENES AND THEIR EFFECTS

Myrcene

> **Effects**: Sedative, relaxing.

Potential Benefits for Cancer: Myrcene is beneficial for cancer patients suffering from sleep disturbances or pain. It is also believed to enhance the permeability of cell membranes, potentially increasing the absorption of cannabinoids.

Limonene

> **Effects**: Mood-enhancing, anti-stress, anti-bacterial, and anti-fungal.

Potential Benefits for Cancer: Limonene may help alleviate depression and anxiety, common issues among cancer patients. Research also suggests limonene has anti-cancer properties, particularly in breast cancer by inducing apoptosis of cancer cells.

Caryophyllene

> **Effects**: Anti-inflammatory, analgesic, and may protect the digestive system.

Potential Benefits for Cancer: Caryophyllene binds to CB2 receptors, which are found mainly in the immune system. This interaction can help reduce inflammation and pain without producing euphoric effects, making it ideal for inflammatory pain management in cancer patients.

Pinene

Effects: Alertness-enhancing, anti-inflammatory, and bronchodilator.

Potential Benefits for Cancer: Pinene can help counteract some of the cognitive impairments associated with THC, improving alertness and memory. Its anti-inflammatory properties are also helpful for managing pain and swelling.

Linalool

Effects: Calming, sedative, and may enhance immune function.

Potential Benefits for Cancer: Linalool can help manage anxiety and insomnia. It also has potential as an adjuvant to enhance the therapeutic effects of certain chemotherapy drugs.

HOW TO CHOOSE MEDICAL CANNABIS BASED ON TERPENES

Identifying Needs: Patients should start by identifying specific symptoms they hope to manage with cannabis, such as pain, insomnia, anxiety, or inflammation.

Consultation with Healthcare Providers: Engaging with a healthcare provider knowledgeable in medical cannabis can provide insights into which terpene profiles may be most effective for their particular needs.

Sourcing Quality Products: Choosing high-quality cannabis products that provide detailed terpene profiles is crucial. Patients should look for products tested by reputable third-party labs that confirm the presence and concentration of specific terpenes.

Experimentation Under Guidance: Due to the subjective nature of cannabis effects, patients might need to experiment with different strains and products under medical guidance to find the one that best suits their needs. Keeping a detailed journal during this process can help track the effectiveness of different terpene profiles.

CONCLUSION

Terpenes play a significant role in the therapeutic potential of cannabis, especially in the context of cancer treatment. By understanding the effects of different terpenes and choosing cannabis strains that align with their specific therapeutic needs, cancer patients can better manage symptoms and improve their quality of life. This knowledge, combined with professional guidance and careful product selection, can lead to a more targeted and effective use of cannabis in cancer care.

METHODS OF CONSUMING CANNABIS MEDICINES: FINDING YOUR FIT

As you explore the potential of cannabis-based therapies in your cancer care, understanding the different methods of consuming these medicines is crucial. Each form has its unique properties, benefits, and considerations, which can significantly impact your experience and the effectiveness of the treatment. This chapter delves into the various cannabis products available on the market, comparing organic options to their non-organic counterparts, helping you choose the best method for your needs.

TRADITIONAL SMOKING

Description: Smoking cannabis is one of the oldest and most immediate methods of consumption. It involves inhaling the smoke from burning cannabis flowers.

Pros:

Rapid onset of effects, providing quick relief.

Easy to dose gradually, as effects are felt almost immediately.

Cons:

Smoking can irritate the lungs and respiratory system, which is not ideal for patients with compromised lung health.

The combustion process can produce harmful byproducts.

Organic vs. Non-Organic: Organic cannabis is grown without synthetic pesticides or fertilizers, which can be crucial for maintaining overall health, especially for cancer patients. Smoking organic cannabis reduces exposure to potentially harmful chemicals that could be present in non-organic products.

VAPORIZATION

Description: Vaporization involves heating cannabis flowers or concentrates just enough to release the active compounds without causing combustion.

Pros:

Healthier than smoking as it reduces the inhalation of tar and carcinogens.

Provides quick relief similar to smoking but is smoother on the lungs.

Cons:

Requires specific equipment, such as a vaporizer.

Can be more costly upfront due to the investment in technology.

Organic vs. Non-Organic: Choosing organic cannabis for vaporization is similarly beneficial as it ensures that you are vaporizing a product free of synthetic additives and pesticides, providing a cleaner experience.

EDIBLES

Description: Cannabis-infused foods and drinks offer an alternative to inhalation methods. The range includes baked goods, gummies, chocolates, and beverages.

Pros:

Provides prolonged effects that can last several hours, beneficial for ongoing relief.

Avoids respiratory exposure, suitable for patients with lung or throat issues.

Cons:

Delayed onset of effects, which can lead to overconsumption if not carefully dosed.

Effects can be unpredictable depending on individual digestion and metabolism.

Organic vs. Non-Organic: Organic edibles ensure that all ingredients, including the cannabis extract, are free from harmful chemicals and additives, promoting a healthier option for patients.

TINCTURES

Description: Tinctures are alcohol-based cannabis extracts taken sublingually (under the tongue). They are also available in oil-based forms which can be swallowed or added to food.

Pros:

> More controlled dosing than smoking or vaporizing.
>
> Faster onset than edibles but longer-lasting than inhalation.

Cons:

> Can have an unpleasant taste that might require dilution with other fluids.
>
> Dosage needs to be measured carefully to avoid too strong effects.

Organic vs. Non-Organic: Organic tinctures are preferable as they ensure that the extraction process hasn't introduced any residual solvents or pesticides, maintaining the purity and potency of the cannabis.

TOPICALS

Description: Cannabis-infused creams, balms, and lotions are applied directly to the skin. Ideal for localized relief.

Pros:

> Targeted relief to specific areas of the body.

> Non-psychoactive, regardless of THC content.

Cons:

> Effects are limited to the area of application and do not address systemic symptoms.

> Absorption rates can vary significantly between individuals.

Organic vs. Non-Organic: With topicals, using organic products can be particularly important, as the skin can absorb harmful chemicals present in non-organic cannabis products.

COMPARISON AND CONCLUSION

Choosing between these methods involves considering your health, lifestyle, and specific needs. For cancer patients, methods that provide controlled dosing and avoid respiratory risks, like tinctures and edibles, are often recommended. However, the immediacy of relief required and personal preferences also play significant roles.

Opting for organic cannabis products across all these methods can enhance safety and efficacy, particularly important for those with compromised health due to cancer. By selecting the method that best aligns with your therapeutic goals and personal values, you can integrate cannabis medicine into your treatment plan effectively and safely.

STRAIN SPECIFICS: CANNABIS VARIETIES AND THEIR THERAPEUTIC APPLICATIONS

In the world of medicinal cannabis, understanding the nuances between different strains is crucial for targeting specific ailments and enhancing treatment outcomes. Cannabis strains are not one-size-fits-all; each variety has unique properties, cannabinoid profiles, and terpene compositions that can significantly influence their effects. This chapter delves into the recommended strains for various medical conditions, providing a guide to help patients and healthcare providers choose the most appropriate cannabis for therapeutic purposes.

PHARMAJUANA

PAIN RELIEF: INDICA STRAINS

Strains: Afghan Kush, Granddaddy Purple, Northern Lights

Characteristics: These strains are renowned for their high levels of THC and myrcene terpenes, which contribute to their sedative effects. They are ideal for treating chronic pain and muscle spasms.

Best For: Conditions like arthritis, neuropathy, and fibromyalgia benefit from these strains due to their deep body-relaxing effects.

ANXIETY AND STRESS: HYBRID AND CBD-RICH STRAINS

Strains: ACDC, Cannatonic, Harlequin

Characteristics: These strains typically have a balanced or high CBD to THC ratio, reducing the likelihood of inducing anxiety, a common side effect of THC-dominant strains.

Best For: Patients suffering from anxiety, PTSD, and stress-related disorders find these strains helpful for their calming and uplifting effects without a strong psychoactive high.

DEPRESSION: SATIVA STRAINS

Strains: Jack Herer, Sour Diesel, Super Lemon Haze

Characteristics: Known for their uplifting and energizing effects, these sativa-dominant strains are high in THC and terpenes like limonene and pinene that can boost mood and energy.

Best For: Their euphoric and activating properties make them suitable for daytime use, especially in treating depression and fatigue.

NAUSEA AND APPETITE STIMULATION: THC-DOMINANT STRAINS

Strains: OG Kush, Pineapple Express, Chemdawg

Characteristics: These strains are high in THC, which is proven to help reduce nausea and stimulate appetite, making them valuable for patients undergoing chemotherapy.

Best For: Cancer patients and those with eating disorders such as anorexia can benefit from the antiemetic and appetite-boosting effects of these strains.

INSOMNIA AND SLEEP DISORDERS: INDICA-DOMINANT STRAINS

Strains: Bubba Kush, Purple Kush, Blue Cheese

PHARMAJUANA

Characteristics: Rich in sedative terpenes like myrcene and linalool, these indica strains are effective for promoting relaxation and sleep.

Best For: Patients with insomnia, sleep apnea, or restless leg syndrome will find these strains help in achieving a more restful sleep.

NEUROLOGICAL DISORDERS: HIGH-CBD STRAINS

Strains: Charlotte's Web, Ringo's Gift, Harle-Tsu

Characteristics: These strains are particularly high in CBD and low in THC, suitable for treating conditions without psychoactive effects.

Best For: Effective in treating epilepsy, multiple sclerosis, and Parkinson's disease, these strains provide relief from seizures, spasms, and pain without significant intoxication.

INFLAMMATORY CONDITIONS: BALANCED CBD/THC STRAINS

Strains: Sweet and Sour Widow, Stephen Hawking Kush, Cannatonic

Characteristics: These strains offer a balance of CBD and THC, providing anti-inflammatory benefits and pain relief with mild psychoactive effects.

Best For: Conditions like Crohn's disease, rheumatoid arthritis, and inflammatory bowel disease benefit from the anti-inflammatory properties of these balanced strains.

CONCLUSION: A STRAIN FOR EVERY PAIN

The diversity in cannabis strains allows for tailored treatments that can more precisely address specific symptoms and conditions. By selecting a strain whose profile aligns with their particular medical needs, patients can optimize their therapeutic outcomes. This guide serves as a starting point for conversations between patients and their healthcare providers about incorporating medicinal cannabis into their treatment plans. As the body of research grows and as more clinical trials are conducted, the understanding of specific strain effects will continue to evolve, further refining the use of cannabis in medical treatment.

Below is a simplified version of a chart which focuses on common types of cancer and the general characteristics of cannabis strains or cannabinoids thought to be beneficial for each.

Type of Cancer	Recommended Cannabis Type	Key Benefits
Breast Cancer	CBD-dominant strains	Anti-inflammatory, may help reduce tumor growth, pain relief
Lung Cancer	THC/CBD balanced strains	Pain relief, appetite stimulation, anti-emetic
Prostate Cancer	High CBD strain	Anti-proliferative, potential to inhibit tumor growth
Colorectal Cancer	THC-dominant strains	Pain management, nausea control, appetite stimulation
Leukemia	High THC strains	Potential to induce apoptosis in cancer cells, pain relief
Pancreatic Cancer	THC/CBD balanced strains	Anti-inflammatory, anti-cancer properties, pain management
Ovarian Cancer	CBD-dominant strains	Pain relief, may help reduce inflammation and tumor growth

Type of Cancer	Recommended Cannabis Type	Key Benefits
Brain Cancer (e.g., Gliomas)	THC and CBD combination	Anti-tumor effects, help with reducing seizures, neuroprotection
Skin Cancer	Topical CBD and THC products	Direct application to tumor sites, pain relief, reduce inflammation

EXPLANATION:

CBD-dominant strains are often recommended for their anti-inflammatory and anti-proliferative properties without significant psychoactive effects, making them suitable for patients concerned about the "high" associated with THC.

THC-dominant strains are valued for their potent pain-relieving properties and their ability to help manage nausea and stimulate appetite, particularly beneficial in combating the side effects of chemotherapy.

THC/CBD balanced strains offer a combination of psychoactive and therapeutic benefits, potentially enhancing the properties of each through the entourage effect. These strains can provide a balance between effective symptom management and minimal psychoactive effects.

Topical products containing THC and CBD can be beneficial for skin cancer, as they allow patients to apply cannabinoids directly to the affected area, potentially reducing tumor growth and relieving local pain and inflammation.

NOTE:

The use of cannabis for cancer treatment should always be guided by a healthcare professional knowledgeable in both oncology and medical cannabis. This chart provides a general overview and should not replace professional medical advice. The effectiveness and suitability of specific cannabis strains or products can vary based on individual patient conditions, other ongoing treatments, and personal health considerations.

INTEGRATING CANNABIS WITH CANCER TREATMENTS: GUIDELINES ON DOSING AND ADMINISTRATION

As the use of cannabis in cancer care continues to gain acceptance, understanding how to integrate it effectively with traditional cancer treatments like chemotherapy and radiation is crucial. This chapter provides insights into the potential interactions between cannabis and other cancer therapies, alongside practical guidelines for dosing and administration.

INTEGRATING CANNABIS WITH TRADITIONAL CANCER TREATMENTS

Chemotherapy and Cannabis:

Synergistic Effects: Some studies suggest that cannabis can enhance the effectiveness of certain chemotherapy agents by increasing cancer cell susceptibility to chemotherapy-induced death.

Managing Side Effects: Cannabis is particularly valued for its ability to manage side effects associated with chemotherapy, such as nausea, vomiting, and loss of appetite.

Timing and Coordination: It's important to coordinate the timing of cannabis use with chemotherapy cycles. Discussing this with your healthcare provider will ensure that cannabis use is complementary and not interfering with the chemotherapeutic agents.

Radiation and Cannabis:

Radioprotective Effects: Preliminary research indicates that certain cannabinoids may have radioprotective properties that can help protect healthy cells during radiation therapy.

Enhancing Comfort: Cannabis may also help manage pain and inflammation caused by radiation therapy, improving patient comfort and potentially adherence to treatment schedules.

Important Considerations:

Interaction Risks: While cannabis is generally safe, it can interact with some medications. Always consult with your oncologist to ensure there are no adverse interactions with your specific cancer treatments.

Clinical Guidance: As cannabis research evolves, ongoing communication with healthcare providers is essential to safely integrate cannabis into your cancer treatment plan.

DOSING AND ADMINISTRATION

Dosing Guidelines:

Starting Low and Going Slow: Begin with a low dose, especially if you are new to cannabis or have concerns about its psychoactive effects. For THC-containing products, this might mean starting with as little as 2.5 mg of THC.

CBD Considerations: If using CBD-dominant products, higher initial doses (such as 20-25 mg) can be appropriate, as CBD does not cause psychoactive effects and is well-tolerated even at higher doses.

Titration Methods:

Incremental Adjustments: Gradually adjust the dose based on your response. Increases should be small and given adequate time (days to weeks) to assess effects. This is crucial to avoid overmedication and to pinpoint the optimal dose for symptom relief.

Monitoring Effects: Keep a detailed log of your cannabis use, including type, dose, time of administration, and effects. This record will help your healthcare provider make informed adjustments.

ROUTES OF ADMINISTRATION:

Inhalation (Smoking/Vaping): Offers quick onset of effects, which can be helpful for acute symptom management but more challenging to dose precisely.

Oral (Edibles, Capsules): Provides longer-lasting effects with a delayed onset, beneficial for sustained symptom control. Requires careful dosing due to the intensity and duration of effects.

Sublingual (Tinctures, Sprays): Offers a middle ground with a faster onset than edibles but more controlled dosing than inhalation.

Topical (Creams, Balms): Useful for localized symptoms like pain and inflammation without systemic effects.

CONCLUSION

Integrating cannabis into your cancer treatment regimen requires thoughtful consideration of the type of treatment, the specific cannabis product, and the most effective dosing strategy. With careful planning and consultation with healthcare providers, cannabis can serve as a valuable adjunct therapy, helping to enhance the efficacy of traditional treatments and manage associated side effects. This approach ensures that you harness the benefits of cannabis safely and effectively, tailored to your individual needs and treatment goals.

SAFETY AND SIDE EFFECTS: NAVIGATING CANNABIS USE IN CANCER CARE

While cannabis offers numerous benefits for cancer patients, like any therapeutic agent, it is not without its risks. Understanding the safety concerns and potential side effects associated with cannabis use is crucial for minimizing risks and maximizing benefits. This chapter outlines the common side effects, long-term risks, and contraindications of cannabis use in cancer care.

COMMON SIDE EFFECTS

Psychoactive Effects:

THC-Induced: The most well-known side effect of cannabis, particularly strains or products high in THC, is its psychoactive impact. Users may experience changes in mood, impaired short-term memory, altered sense of time, and sensory perception. These **effects are generally temporary but can be unsettling for new users.**

Managing Psychoactivity: Opting for strains with lower THC and higher CBD ratios can mitigate some of these psychoactive effects. Additionally, careful dosing and gradual titration can help manage these responses.

Physical Side Effects:

Dry Mouth and Eyes: Commonly known as "cottonmouth," this side effect occurs due to cannabis's influence on salivary glands. Eye dryness or redness can also occur.

Dizziness: Particularly after consuming high-THC cannabis, some individuals may experience dizziness due to a temporary drop in blood pressure.

Coordination and Reaction Time: THC can impair motor skills and reaction time, making it unsafe to drive or operate heavy machinery while under the influence.

Digestive Issues:

Nausea and Vomiting: Ironically, while cannabis is often used to reduce chemotherapy-induced nausea, in some cases, especially with high doses, it can induce nausea and vomiting.

Changes in Appetite: While often seen as a benefit, the appetite-stimulating effects of THC can lead to unintended weight gain.

LONG-TERM RISKS

Cognitive Effects:

Memory and Cognition: Long-term, heavy use of high-THC cannabis has been linked to subtle impairments in memory, cognition, and attention. These effects are typically more pronounced in individuals who start using cannabis at a young age.

Mental Health:

Mood Disorders: Long-term use can affect mental health, potentially exacerbating symptoms of existing conditions such as depression or bipolar disorder.

Cannabis Use Disorder: Chronic use can lead to dependence, characterized by the inability to stop using cannabis despite it causing health and social issues.

CONTRAINDICATIONS

Psychiatric Conditions:

Psychosis and Schizophrenia: Individuals with schizophrenia, or who are at high risk of psychosis, should avoid high-THC cannabis, as it can exacerbate symptoms or trigger new episodes.

Severe Anxiety or Panic Disorders: While some patients use cannabis to alleviate anxiety, high-THC products can sometimes induce anxiety or panic attacks in susceptible individuals.

Substance Use Disorders:

History of Substance Abuse: Patients with a history of substance abuse may be at higher risk for developing cannabis use disorder.

Medical supervision is crucial to monitor and manage use appropriately.

Cardiovascular Health:

Heart Disease: Cannabis can increase heart rate and affect blood pressure, posing risks for patients with cardiovascular conditions. Consulting with a healthcare provider is essential before starting cannabis, especially for those with heart-related issues.

CONCLUSION

The decision to use cannabis as part of cancer treatment should be made with full awareness of the potential side effects and risks. It is essential to have open, ongoing conversations with healthcare providers to tailor cannabis use to your specific health needs, ensuring it complements your comprehensive cancer care plan safely and effectively. By understanding and respecting the power of cannabis, patients can better navigate its use to enhance their quality of life during cancer treatment.

GLOBAL BITES: EDIBLE PREPARATIONS OF CANNABIS AROUND THE WORLD

Cannabis has been a part of culinary traditions across the globe for centuries, not only for its psychoactive and medicinal effects but also for its versatility in recipes. This chapter takes you on a culinary tour, showcasing how different cultures incorporate cannabis into edible preparations. From traditional dishes to modern culinary innovations, we explore the diverse ways cannabis is consumed around the world.

BHANG - INDIA

Description: One of the most ancient and culturally significant cannabis edibles is Bhang, used both for its medicinal properties and as a part of religious festivities, particularly during Holi, the festival of colors.

Ingredients: Bhang is typically made from the leaves and buds of cannabis ground into a paste. It's mixed with spices, milk, and sometimes yogurt or nuts to create a potent drink.

Cultural Context: Bhang has been part of Ayurvedic medicine for thousands of years, used to treat ailments such as digestive issues and anxiety.

PHARMAJUANA

MAJOUN - MOROCCO

Description: Majoun is a famous Moroccan cannabis-infused confection, often referred to as "Moroccan candy." It's known for its sweet, fruity flavor and herbal undertones.

Ingredients: Traditionally, majoun is made from cannabis butter, dried fruits, nuts, honey, and a mix of spices including cinnamon and anise.

Cultural Context: Majoun is typically consumed in small quantities due to its potency. It's often associated with hospitality and special occasions.

GANJA TEA - JAMAICA

Description: In Jamaica, cannabis is commonly brewed into a tea which is valued both for its calming effects and its medicinal benefits, especially for morning sickness and rheumatism.

Ingredients: The tea is simple, made by boiling cannabis leaves with water and sometimes adding ginger or other local herbs for flavor.

Cultural Context: Ganja tea is a home remedy used in rural areas, reflecting the Rastafarian spiritual and healing use of cannabis.

PHARMAJUANA

CANNABIS-INFUSED BROWNIES - UNITED STATES

Description: Cannabis-infused brownies are perhaps the most iconic modern edible, popularized by the counterculture movements of the 1960s.

Ingredients: These brownies are made by incorporating cannabis butter or oil into the batter, ensuring even distribution of THC.

Cultural Context: The brownie has become a staple in dispensaries across states where cannabis is legalized, serving as a discreet and easy-to-dose method of consumption.

SPACE CAKES - NETHERLANDS

Description: Space cakes are a popular way to consume cannabis in Amsterdam and across the Netherlands, often found in coffee shops.

Ingredients: They can vary in flavor and ingredients but typically involve mixing cannabis butter into the cake batter.

Cultural Context: The Netherlands has been at the forefront of cannabis legalization in Europe, and space cakes offer both locals and tourists a palatable way to enjoy cannabis.

PHARMAJUANA

HEMP SEED DUMPLINGS - CHINA

Description: Hemp seeds, which do not contain THC, have been used in Chinese cooking for thousands of years. They are noted for their nutritional benefits and are often incorporated into dumplings.

Ingredients: These dumplings are made with hemp seeds ground into a paste, combined with other fillings like pork or vegetables.

Cultural Context: While these dumplings don't offer the psychoactive effects of THC, they highlight the nutritional use of hemp, another important aspect of cannabis.

A DELICIOUS SPECTRUM

These dishes and preparations not only provide a delicious entry into the world of cannabis but also highlight the cultural significance and historical use of this versatile plant. Whether used for its psychoactive properties, medicinal benefits, or nutritional value, cannabis continues to be an integral part of culinary traditions around the world. As we explore these global flavors, we also appreciate the deeper connection between cultures and cannabis, understanding its role in social, spiritual, and medicinal contexts. This chapter invites you to think beyond the herb as just a medicine or a recreational drug but as a bridge between tradition, culture, and community across the globe.

RESEARCH AND DEVELOPMENTS: THE FUTURE OF CANNABIS IN CANCER TREATMENT

Cannabis research has made significant strides, particularly in the field of oncology, where it offers promising prospects for symptom management and potentially as a direct anti-cancer agent. This chapter reviews current research on cannabis in cancer treatment, highlighting key studies and discussing what the future may hold for cannabis medicine in oncology.

CURRENT RESEARCH

Clinical Trials and Studies:

Symptom Management: Numerous studies have validated the efficacy of cannabis, especially cannabinoids like THC and CBD, in managing cancer-related symptoms. These include pain, nausea, and vomiting induced by chemotherapy, as well as improving appetite and sleep.

Anti-Cancer Properties: Research into cannabinoids' ability to kill cancer cells in vitro and in animal models is ongoing, with some studies showing that cannabinoids can induce cell death, inhibit cell growth, and prevent the spread of cancer cells. For example, studies have shown that THC and CBD can induce apoptosis in glioma cells and inhibit the growth of tumors in animal models of glioblastoma.

PHARMAJUANA

The British Journal of Cancer reported findings that cannabinoids might inhibit hormone-sensitive prostate cancer cells.

The Journal of Clinical Oncology has published results from surveys indicating that many oncologists consider cannabis as a potential adjunct to conventional cancer treatments, citing evidence of benefit in symptom management.

FUTURE OUTLOOK

Ongoing Studies:

Precision Medicine: As the field of precision medicine expands, there is growing interest in how specific cannabinoids can target specific types of cancer cells with minimal side effects. This approach aims to tailor treatments to individual genetic profiles, potentially integrating cannabis-based therapies into personalized cancer care plans.

Combination Therapies: Researchers are exploring how combining cannabinoids with traditional cancer treatments like chemotherapy or radiation may enhance efficacy and reduce side effects. Early results are promising, indicating that cannabinoids might make cancer cells more responsive to radiation therapy.

REGULATORY CHANGES AND IMPLICATIONS:

FDA Approvals: The future of cannabis in oncology will likely be influenced by the U.S. Food and Drug Administration (FDA) and similar bodies worldwide as they continue to evaluate cannabis for medical use. Approval of cannabis-based medicines, such as the already FDA-approved cannabinoids for nausea and anorexia associated with cancer treatments, could pave the way for broader acceptance and integration into mainstream medicine.

TECHNOLOGICAL ADVANCES:

Drug Delivery Systems: Innovations in drug delivery systems, such as nanoparticle carriers for cannabinoids, are being developed to improve the bioavailability and targeting of cannabis-based treatments, which could dramatically enhance their effectiveness and reduce side effects.

GLOBAL TRENDS:

International Research Collaborations: Increased global interest in cannabis research is leading to international collaborations, pooling resources, and knowledge to drive discoveries and clinical trial designs that could revolutionize cancer treatment.

CONCLUSION

The intersection of cannabis research and oncology holds a compelling promise for the future of cancer care. Current research underscores the potential of cannabis not only in symptom management but also as a component of direct anti-cancer therapies. As ongoing studies unfold and new technologies emerge, the next decade could see transformative developments in how cannabis is integrated into oncological practices, offering hope and improved outcomes for patients worldwide. This evolving landscape requires continuous monitoring and participation from the medical community to ensure that cannabis-based therapies are safe, effective, and accessible to those who need them most.

BEYOND MEDICINE: THE BROADER BENEFITS OF CANNABIS

While the focus of this book is primarily on the medical applications of cannabis, particularly in the context of cancer treatment, it's worth exploring the plant's additional benefits. Cannabis has a range of uses beyond medicine, encompassing industrial, recreational, and environmental aspects. This chapter highlights these broader applications, offering a more comprehensive view of the plant's versatility and utility.

RECREATIONAL USE

Enhancing Well-Being: Cannabis is widely used for its psychoactive properties, which many people find enhances their sense of well-being. The ability to induce relaxation and reduce anxiety is a significant draw for recreational users, contributing to mental health in settings outside of clinical depression or anxiety treatments.

Social Interaction: Socially, cannabis often plays a role in bonding and community-building activities. Shared experiences around cannabis can foster a sense of camaraderie and community among users.

PHARMAJUANA

INDUSTRIAL HEMP

Fiber and Textiles: Cannabis sativa, particularly the hemp variety, is used for its strong fibers, which are made into a variety of products, including clothing, bags, ropes, and other textiles. Hemp fibers are celebrated for their durability, breathability, and antimicrobial properties.

Building Materials: Hemp is also used in building materials like hempcrete, which is known for its insulation properties, light weight, and sustainability. It provides a lower carbon footprint compared to traditional building materials.

Biodegradable Plastics: Innovations in biodegradable plastic alternatives often incorporate hemp. These hemp-based plastics can decompose naturally, offering an environmentally friendly alternative to petroleum-based plastics.

NUTRITIONAL BENEFITS

Hemp Seeds: Known for their nutritional value, hemp seeds are rich in essential fatty acids, protein, and fiber. They are often used in health foods and can be eaten raw, ground into a meal, sprouted, or made into dried sprout powder. Hemp seeds also contain vitamins and minerals and are used in products like hemp milk, oil, and protein powder.

Culinary Uses: Beyond their health benefits, hemp seeds are also used in cooking for their nutty flavor. They can be added to salads, smoothies, and baked goods, enhancing the nutritional profile of various dishes.

ENVIRONMENTAL IMPACT

Sustainability: Cannabis, especially hemp, plays a significant role in sustainable agriculture. It is a fast-growing crop that requires relatively low amounts of water and pesticides. This makes it an environmentally friendly option for crop rotation and sustainable farming practices.

Soil Health: Hemp is known to improve soil health through phytoremediation, whereby it absorbs contaminants from the soil. This property makes hemp valuable in reclaiming and revitalizing polluted lands.

CONCLUSION

The benefits of cannabis extend well beyond its use as a medicine. From recreational and social uses to industrial applications and environmental benefits, cannabis proves to be a versatile plant with a wide range of uses. Understanding these additional benefits can deepen our appreciation of cannabis, highlighting its potential as a multifaceted resource that can contribute to various aspects of life and industry. By embracing the full spectrum of cannabis's applications, we can better advocate for its integration into society, not only as a medical resource but as a valuable commodity in our quest for sustainability and improved quality of life.

ABOUT THE AUTHOR

Dr. Sunayana Pandé is a celebrated minister, naturopathic doctor, metaphysician, and transformational therapist. Her extensive academic background spans psychology, neuroscience, religion, and metaphysics, grounding her as a luminary in her field. As a proud Brahmin Hindu from the Himalayan foothills, Dr. Pandé carries forward a profound lineage, integrating deep spiritual insights with cutting-edge therapeutic approaches.

Dr. Pandé is the visionary author of "Beyond Binary", "Sail Beyond Trauma", and "Life in the Bliss Lane," works that reflect her commitment to transcending traditional narratives. "Beyond Binary" delves into the fluidity of gender and identity, offering transformative insights that challenge societal norms. "Sail Beyond Trauma" introduces readers to her groundbreaking Kappal Otti trauma therapy, which is a pioneering approach designed to navigate and heal the turbulent waters of psychological trauma. "Life in the Bliss Lane" is a guide to wellness, self-love, and joy.

Additionally, as the founder of a unique temple dedicated to Ardhanarishwara, Dr. Pandé provides a sanctuary for non-binary persons, transgender individuals, and drag performers, especially those affected by oppressive legislation. This space not only serves as a religious haven but also as a center for community and spiritual rejuvenation.

In her professional practice, Dr. Pandé employs her innovative autism paradigm, which redefines the therapeutic landscape for neurodiversity. Her health and fitness plans are inclusively crafted, catering specifically to the needs of disabled persons, underscoring her philosophy that wellness should be accessible to all.

Dr. Pandé's activism and advocacy are integral to her identity. Through her work, she endeavors to crack open the conventional frameworks of thinking, fostering new ways for individuals to interact with the world around them and within themselves. Her teachings inspire a wave of change, encouraging others to evolve beyond the confines of their conditioning.

Dr. Sunayana Pandé continues to educate, inspire, and lead, touching the lives of many through her books, therapeutic practices, and dedicated activism.